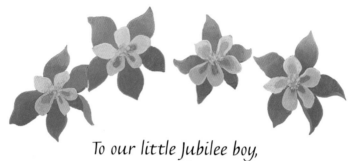

To our little Jubilee boy,
Frankie

LITTLE TIGER PRESS
An imprint of Magi Publications
1 The Coda Centre, 189 Munster Road, London SW6 6AW
www.littletigerpress.com

First published in Great Britain 2003
This edition published 2005

Text and illustrations copyright © Catherine Walters 2003
Catherine Walters has asserted her right to be
identified as the author and illustrator of this work
under the Copyright, Designs and Patents Act, 1988

ISBN 1 84506 347 3
Printed in China
2 4 6 8 10 9 7 5 3 1

Time to Sleep, Alfie Bear!

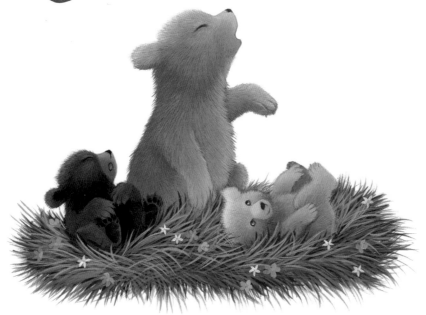

Catherine Walters

LITTLE TIGER PRESS
London

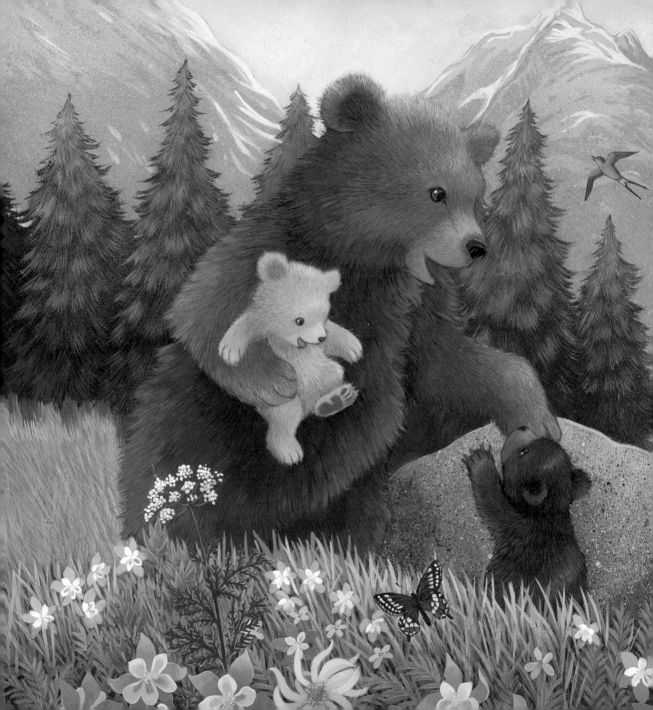

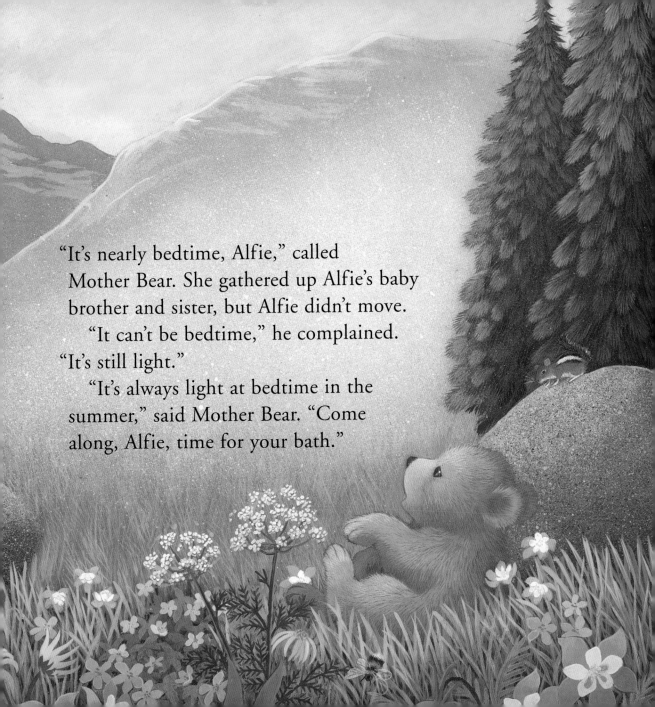

"It's nearly bedtime, Alfie," called
Mother Bear. She gathered up Alfie's baby
brother and sister, but Alfie didn't move.
    "It can't be bedtime," he complained.
"It's still light."
    "It's always light at bedtime in the
summer," said Mother Bear. "Come
along, Alfie, time for your bath."

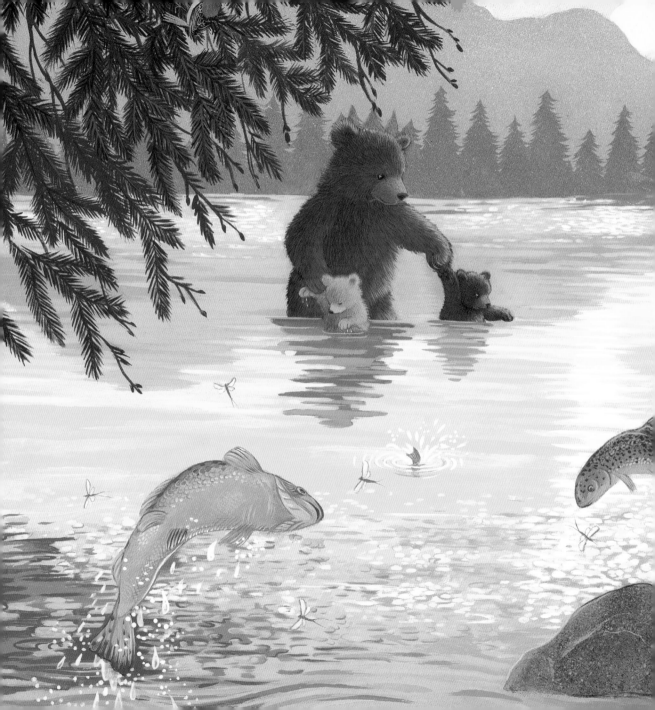

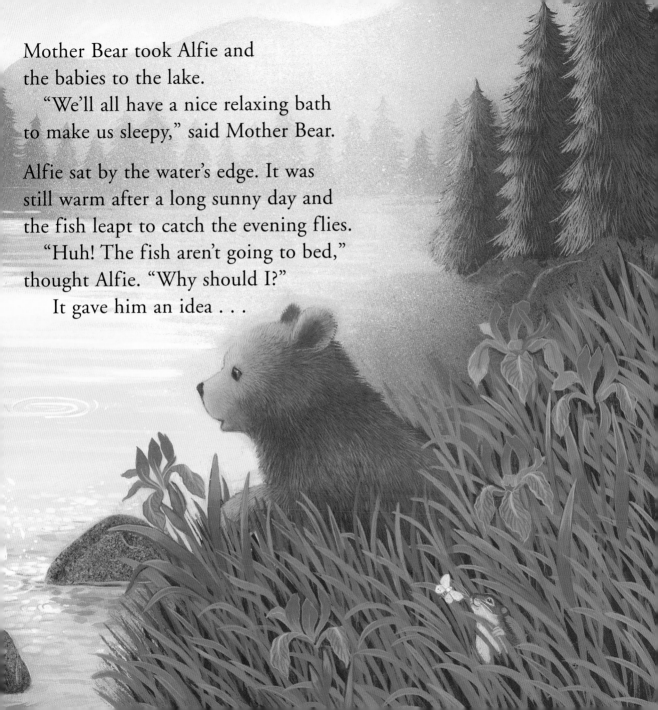

Mother Bear took Alfie and
the babies to the lake.

"We'll all have a nice relaxing bath
to make us sleepy," said Mother Bear.

Alfie sat by the water's edge. It was
still warm after a long sunny day and
the fish leapt to catch the evening flies.

"Huh! The fish aren't going to bed,"
thought Alfie. "Why should I?"

It gave him an idea . . .

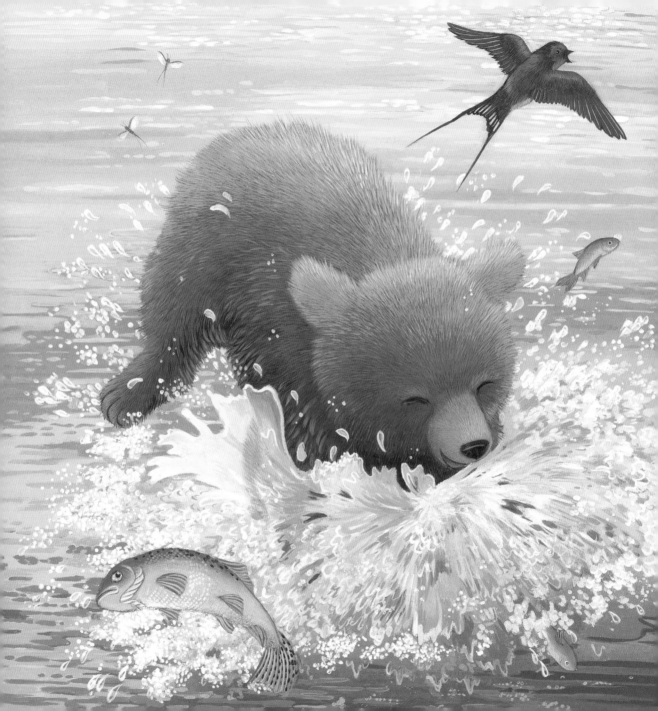

"Look, Mother Bear," shouted Alfie.
"I don't have to go to bed! I'm a fish!"

He began to jump and dive and splash.
The babies loved it. They laughed and
splashed too.

"Don't do that," sighed Mother Bear.
"The babies are getting too excited.
They'll never go to sleep."

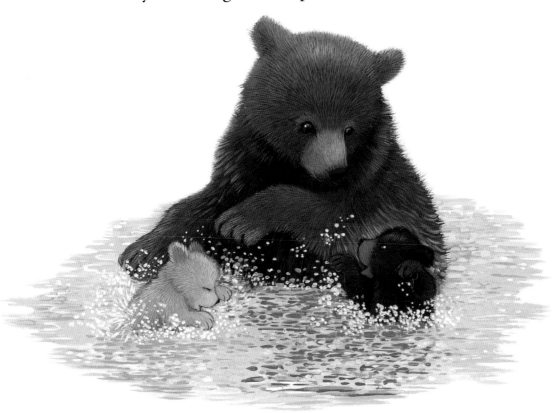

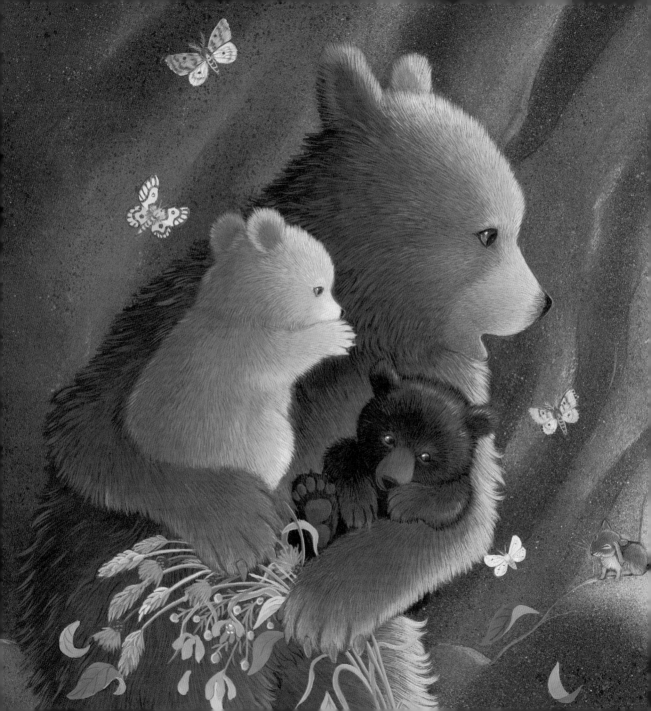

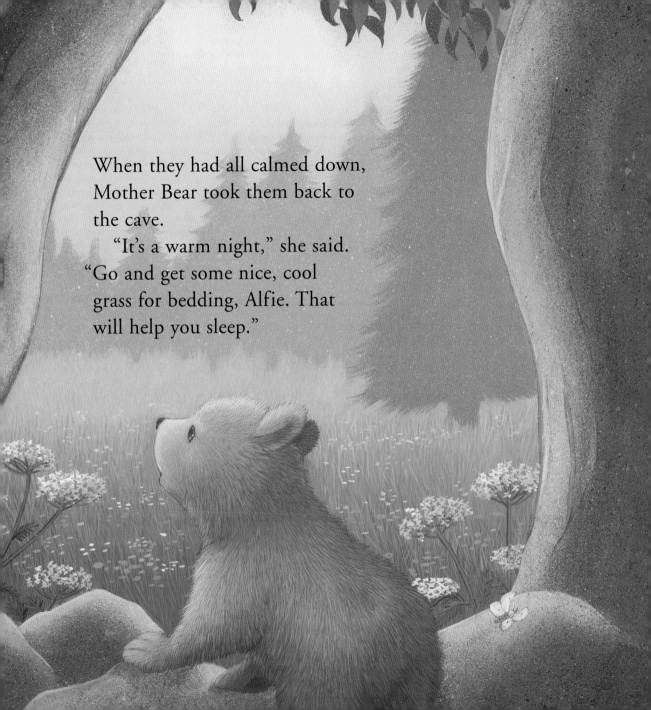

When they had all calmed down,
Mother Bear took them back to
the cave.

"It's a warm night," she said.
"Go and get some nice, cool
grass for bedding, Alfie. That
will help you sleep."

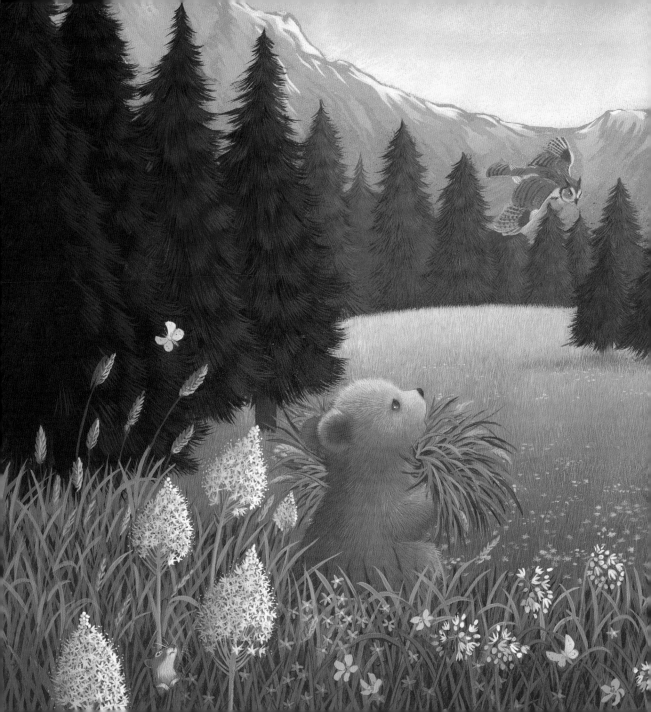

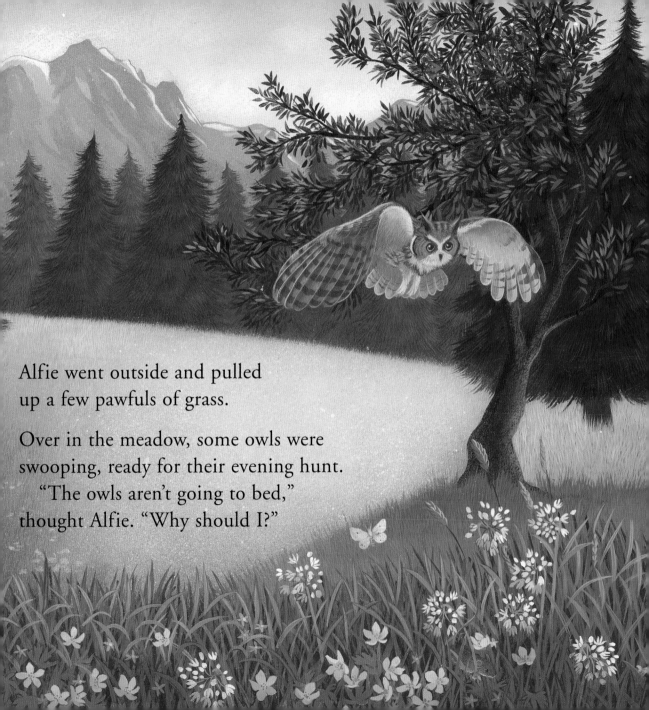

Alfie went outside and pulled
up a few pawfuls of grass.

Over in the meadow, some owls were
swooping, ready for their evening hunt.
   "The owls aren't going to bed,"
thought Alfie. "Why should I?"

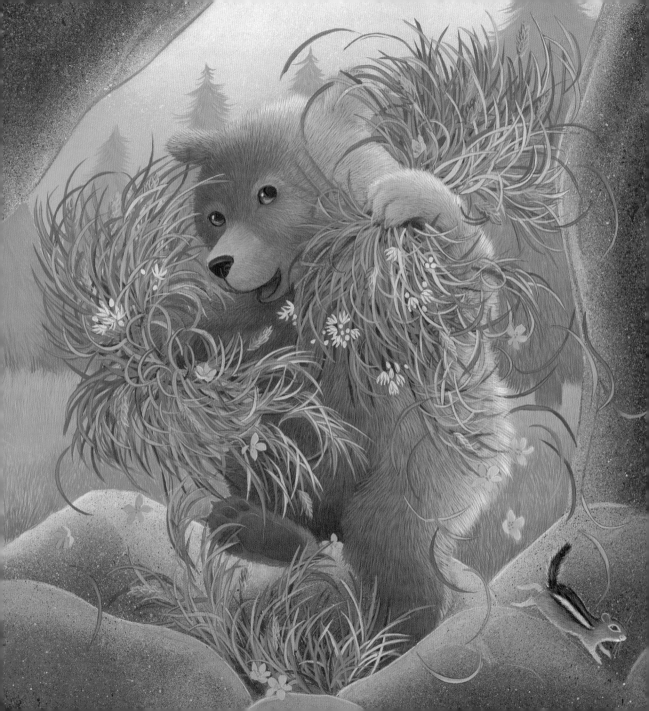

Alfie rushed back into the cave and began to flap his arms. Grass flew everywhere.

"Look! I'm an owl!" he hooted. "I don't need to go to bed. I'm just getting up!"

"Oh Alfie, stop that!" groaned Mother Bear. "Look, the babies are throwing all their lovely bedding around, too. None of you will have anywhere to sleep."

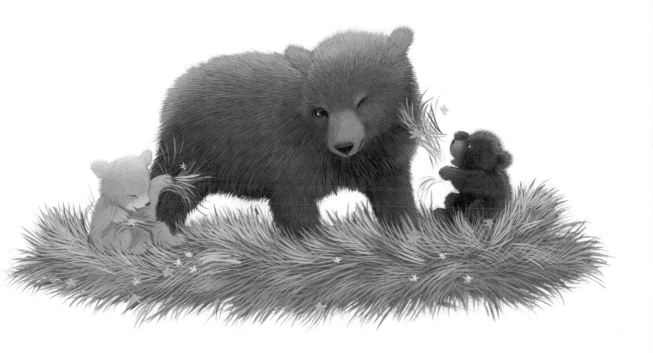

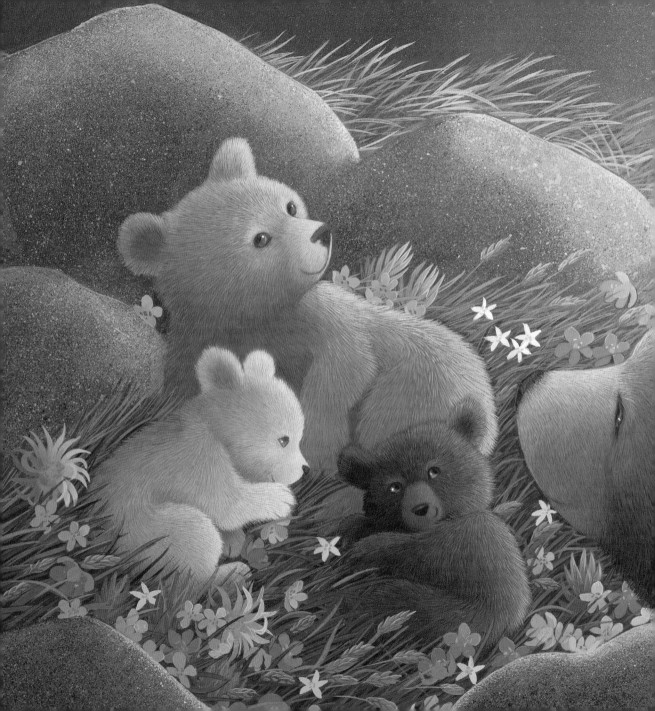

At last, Alfie and the babies were safely
in bed but still they didn't go to sleep.
"I think you need a nice, gentle song,"
said Mother Bear. "Now, close your eyes."
Alfie wasn't listening. Outside, he
could hear wolves howling.
"The wolves aren't going to sleep,"
he thought. "Why should I?"

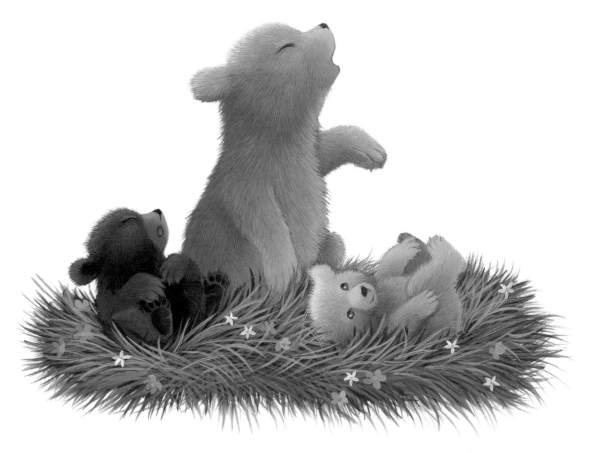

"Look, I'm a wolf! AAAAOOOW!" said Alfie.

"OW, OW, OW!" shrieked the babies, kicking their feet.

Mother Bear wasn't pleased. "That's enough, Alfie," she growled. "I don't want any little wolves in the cave. You can wait outside until the babies are asleep."

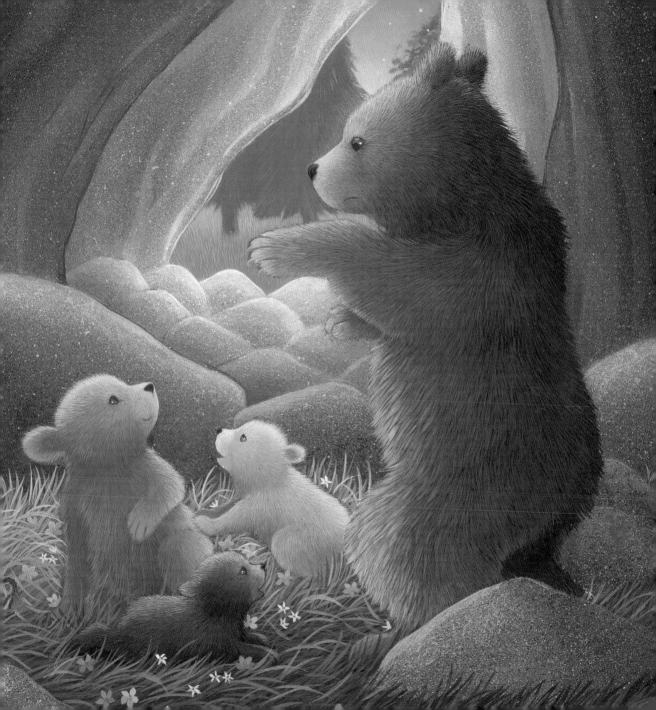

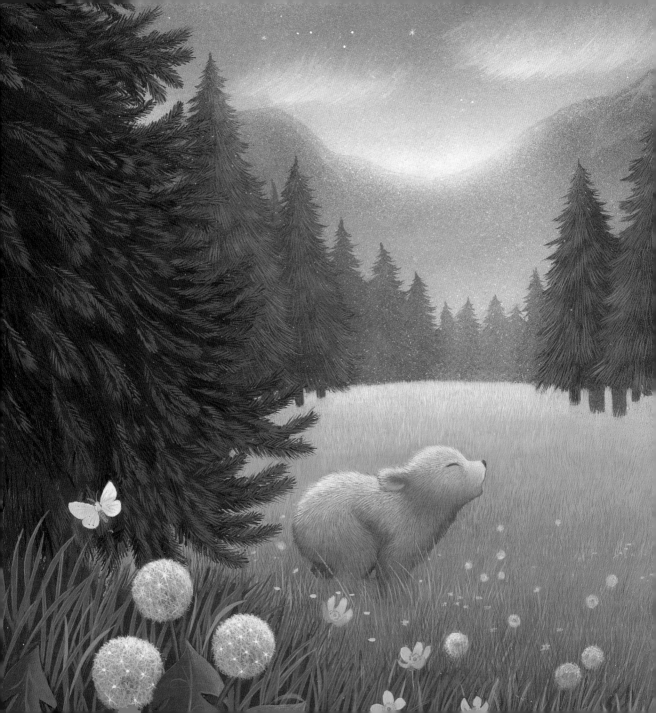

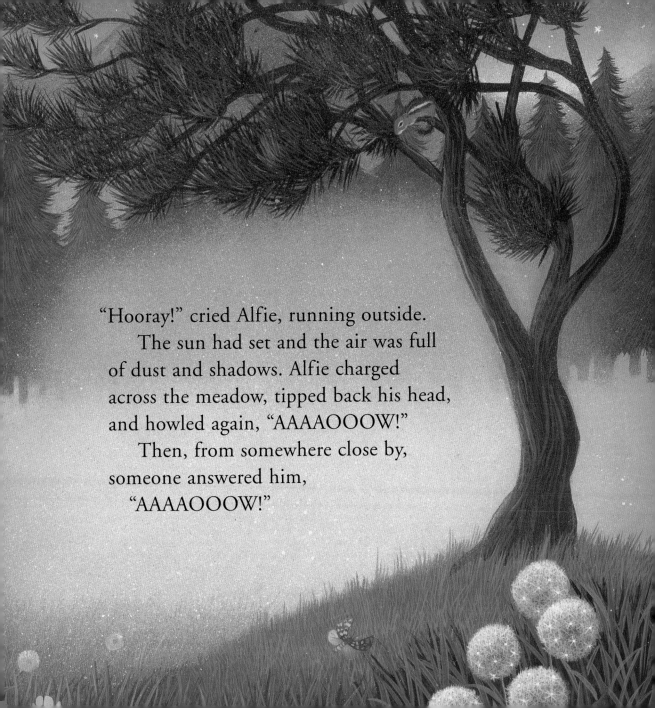

"Hooray!" cried Alfie, running outside.
The sun had set and the air was full
of dust and shadows. Alfie charged
across the meadow, tipped back his head,
and howled again, "AAAAOOOW!"
Then, from somewhere close by,
someone answered him,
"AAAAOOOW!"

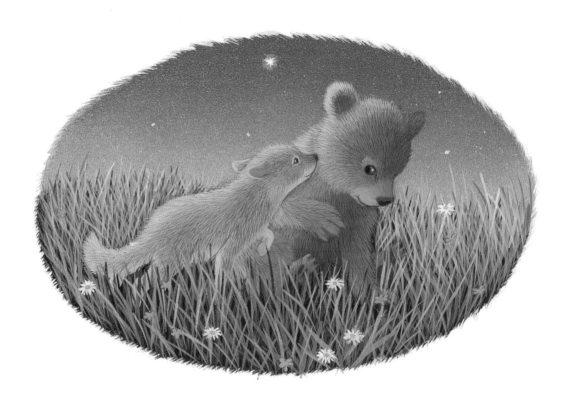

Alfie jumped. There in front of him was
a wolf cub, with his family close by.

The cub sniffed him all over.

"Are you a wolf?" it asked. "You sound
like one, but you don't look like one."

"All little wolf cubs should be in bed
by now," growled Mother Wolf.

"Are you sure you're a wolf?" called
a big, gruff voice . . .

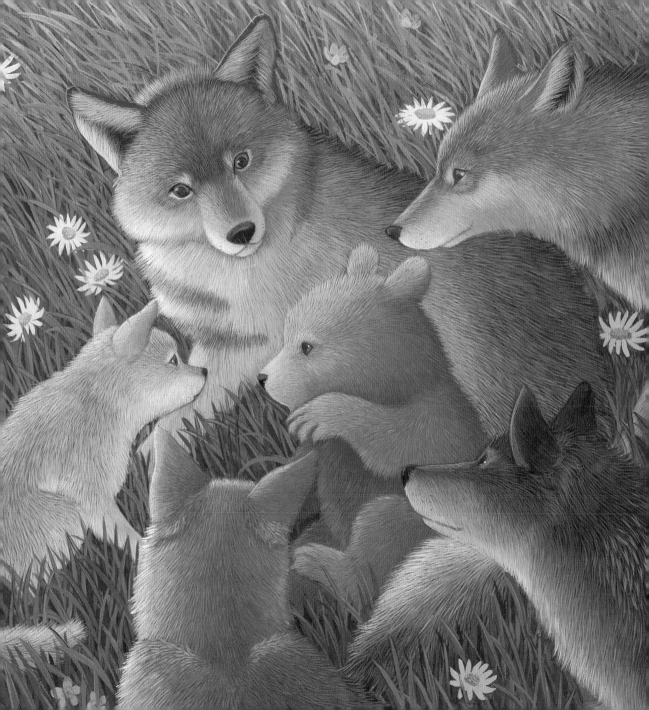

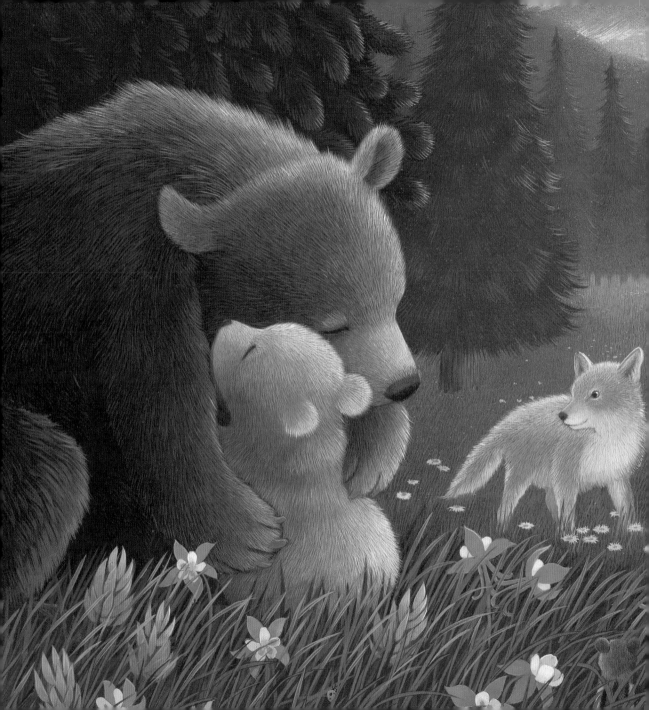

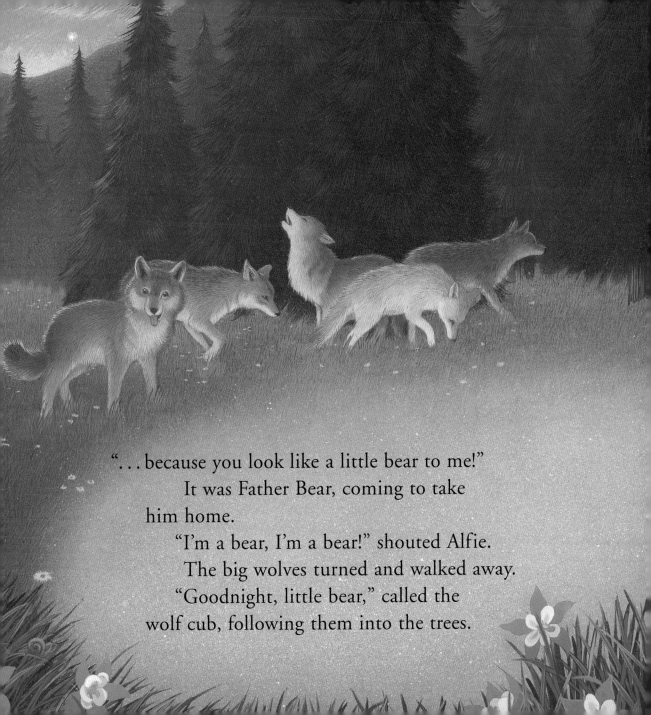

"...because you look like a little bear to me!"
It was Father Bear, coming to take
him home.
"I'm a bear, I'm a bear!" shouted Alfie.
The big wolves turned and walked away.
"Goodnight, little bear," called the
wolf cub, following them into the trees.

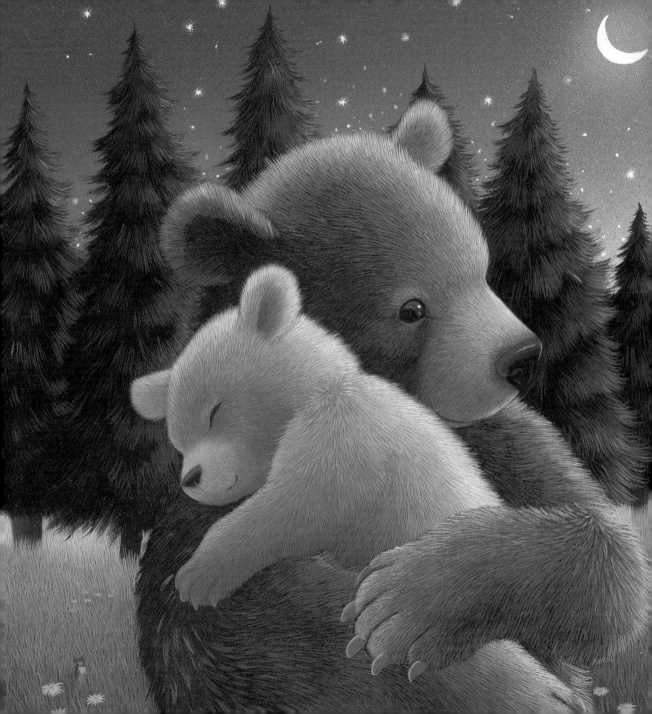

Father Bear snuggled Alfie into his fur.

"So you're a bear?" he said. "But are you a sleepy bear all ready for bed?"

Night had fallen, and the sky sparkled with stars.

"No," said Alfie. "I'm not –"

But before he could finish speaking, he had fallen fast asleep.

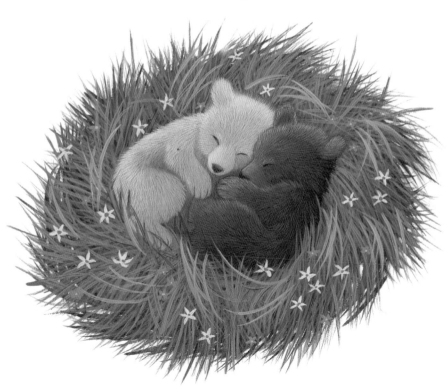